The Handbook for Understanding and Managing Addiction

What is Addiction?

Addiction is a chronic brain disorder characterized by compulsive engagement in rewarding stimuli despite adverse consequences. It is considered a disease because it involves changes to the brain's structure and function, which can lead to a loss of control over the behavior in question.

Addiction can take many forms, including substance addiction (such as to alcohol, drugs, or nicotine) and behavioral addiction (such as to gambling, sex, or shopping). The defining feature of addiction is the continued use of a substance or engagement in a behavior despite negative consequences.

When someone is addicted, they have a strong desire or craving to engage in the behavior, and may experience withdrawal symptoms if they try to stop. They may also develop a tolerance, meaning they need more of the substance or behavior to achieve the same effects.

Addiction can have a wide range of negative effects on an individual's physical and mental health, as well as their relationships, finances, and overall well-being. It is a complex condition that is influenced by a variety of factors including genetics, environment, and personal history.

It's important to note that addiction is not a choice or a moral failing, but a chronic medical condition which can be treated

with professional help, support, and the
right tools.

Types of Addiction

There are various types of addiction, which can be broadly classified into two categories: substance addiction and behavioral addiction.

Substance addiction: This type of addiction occurs when an individual becomes physically and/or psychologically dependent on a substance such as drugs, alcohol, or nicotine. Some examples of substance addiction include:

Alcohol addiction: characterized by excessive drinking that leads to problems with physical and mental health, as well as social and occupational functioning.

Drug addiction: characterized by excessive use of drugs such as opioids, cocaine, marijuana, and amphetamines, which can lead to physical dependence, withdrawal symptoms, and a range of negative effects on health and well-being.

Nicotine addiction: characterized by the compulsive use of tobacco products, which can lead to physical dependence and withdrawal symptoms when an individual tries to quit.

Behavioral addiction: This type of addiction occurs when an individual becomes compulsively engaged in a behavior such as gambling, shopping, sex, or internet use, despite negative consequences. Some examples of behavioral addiction include:

Gambling addiction: characterized by excessive gambling that leads to problems with finances, relationships, and mental health.

Shopping addiction: characterized by excessive shopping that leads to problems with finances and relationships.

Sex addiction: characterized by compulsive sexual behaviors that lead to problems with relationships and mental health.

Internet addiction: characterized by excessive internet use that leads to problems with relationships, occupational functioning, and mental health.

It's worth to note that addiction can often manifest as a combination of substance and behavioral addiction, this condition is known as "co-occurring disorder" or "dual diagnosis". For example, an individual may be addicted to both alcohol and gambling, or drugs and internet use.

It's also important to note that addiction is a complex condition that can manifest differently in different individuals, and that there may be overlap between different types of addiction.

The Impact of Addiction on Individuals and Society

Addiction can have a significant impact on individuals and society, both in terms of physical and mental health, as well as social and economic well-being.

Physical health: Addiction can lead to a range of physical health problems, including organ damage, chronic diseases, and increased risk of injury and death. For example, alcohol and drug addiction can lead to liver damage, heart disease, and increased risk of overdose, while smoking addiction can lead to lung cancer and other respiratory problems. Behavioral addiction such as internet addiction can lead to physical problems such as back pain, carpal tunnel syndrome, and eye strain.

Mental health: Addiction can also have a significant impact on mental health, leading to a range of mental health disorders such as depression, anxiety, and psychosis. For example, individuals with alcohol addiction may experience depression and anxiety, while individuals with drug addiction may experience psychosis and other mental health problems. Behavioral addiction can also lead to mental health disorders such as depression and anxiety.

Social and economic well-being: Addiction can also have a significant impact on social and economic well-being, leading to problems with relationships, employment, and finances. For example, addiction can lead to job loss, financial problems, and strain on relationships, as well as an increased risk of homelessness and poverty. Addiction can also lead to legal problems, such as arrest and incarceration.

Societal impact: Addiction also has a significant impact on society as a whole. The costs of addiction in terms of healthcare, criminal justice, and lost productivity are staggering. Additionally, addiction can lead to increased crime, homelessness, and poverty, which can further strain societal resources.

It's important to note that addiction is a complex and multifaceted condition that can impact individuals in different ways and to different extents. It's also important to note that addiction can be a vicious cycle that can be difficult to break without professional help, support and the right tools.

Understanding the Causes of Addiction

Biological Factors Causing Addiction

There are various biological factors that can contribute to the development of addiction, including genetics, brain chemistry, and changes in the brain's structure and function.

Genetics: Studies have shown that addiction can run in families, suggesting that there is a genetic component to the development of addiction. Researchers have identified specific genes that may increase an individual's risk of developing addiction, but it's important to note that genetics are not the only factor, and that addiction is a complex disorder that is influenced by many factors.

Brain chemistry: Addiction is closely linked to changes in brain chemistry, particularly in the areas of the brain that are involved in reward, motivation, and memory. When an individual uses a substance or engages in a behavior that is addictive, it triggers the release of chemicals in the brain such as dopamine, which leads to feelings of pleasure and euphoria. Over time, the brain can become accustomed to these elevated levels of dopamine and other chemicals, leading to a need for more of the substance or behavior to achieve the same effects.

Brain structure and function: Addiction can lead to changes in the brain's structure and function, particularly in the areas that are involved in decision-making, impulse control, and memory. Research has shown that chronic substance use can lead to changes in the brain's white matter, which can affect communication between different regions of the brain, and can impair decision-making and impulse control.

It's important to note that these biological factors can interact with other factors such as environment, personal history, and mental health conditions to influence the development of addiction. Also, that not all individuals who are exposed to the same risk factors will develop addiction, and that addiction is a complex disorder that is influenced by many factors.

Psychological Factors Causing Addiction

There are various psychological factors that can contribute to the development of addiction, including stress, trauma, and mental health conditions.

Stress: Stress can be a significant risk factor for addiction, as individuals may turn to substances or behaviors as a way to cope with stress and negative emotions. Chronic stress can also lead to changes in brain chemistry and structure, which can increase the risk of addiction.

Trauma: Trauma, such as physical, emotional, or sexual abuse, can also increase the risk of addiction. Trauma can lead to changes in brain chemistry and structure, as well as emotional and mental health problems, which can increase the risk of addiction.

Mental health conditions: Mental health conditions such as depression, anxiety, and PTSD can also increase the risk of addiction. These conditions can lead to changes in brain chemistry and structure, as well as emotional and mental health problems, which can increase the risk of addiction.

Low self-esteem or poor self-worth: Individuals who have poor self-esteem, low self-worth, or feelings of inadequacy may be more likely to turn to substances or behaviors as a way to cope with these feelings.

Life events: Life events such as unemployment, loss of a loved one, or relationship problems, can increase the risk of addiction. These events can lead to stress and emotional distress, which can increase the risk of addiction.

Social factors: Social factors such as peer pressure, cultural influences, and easy access to addictive substances or behaviors can also contribute to the development of addiction.

It's important to note that these psychological factors can interact with other factors such as biology, environment, and personal history to influence the development of addiction. Also, that not all individuals who are exposed to the same risk factors will develop addiction, and that addiction is a complex disorder that is influenced by many factors.

Bleeding can be a serious emergency, and prompt first aid is essential to prevent excessive blood loss and to preserve life.

Social and Environmental Factors Causing Addiction

There are various social and environmental factors that can contribute to the development of addiction, including family dynamics, cultural influences, and access to substances or behaviors.

Family dynamics: Family dynamics can play a significant role in the development of addiction. For example, a family history of addiction can increase an individual's risk of developing addiction, as can growing up in a household where substance abuse or addictive behaviors are present. Additionally, poor communication, lack of emotional support, and high levels of conflict within a family can also increase the risk of addiction.

Cultural influences: Cultural influences can also play a role in the development of addiction. For example, cultural norms around substance use and addiction can vary widely, and an individual's cultural background can influence their risk of developing addiction. Additionally, cultural influences can also affect the types of substances or behaviors to which an individual is exposed, and the level of stigma associated with addiction within a particular culture.

Access to substances or behaviors: Access to substances or behaviors that are addictive can also increase the risk of addiction. For example, easy access to drugs or alcohol, or proximity to gambling venues can increase the risk of addiction.

Additionally, the availability and marketing of certain substances and behaviors can also influence an individual's risk of developing addiction.

Socio-economic status: Socio-economic status can also play a role in the development of addiction. For example, individuals from lower socio-economic backgrounds may be more likely to develop addiction, due to factors such as poverty, lack of education, and limited access to healthcare and other resources.

Trauma and Adverse Childhood Experiences (ACEs): Trauma and Adverse Childhood Experiences (ACEs) can also increase the risk of addiction. Trauma and ACEs can lead to emotional and mental health problems, which can increase the risk of addiction.

It's important to note that these social and environmental factors can interact with other factors such as biology, psychology, and personal history to influence the development of addiction. Also, that not all individuals who are exposed to the same risk factors will develop addiction, and that addiction is a complex disorder that is influenced by many factors.

Identifying and Assessing Addiction

Signs and Symptoms

The signs and symptoms of addiction can vary depending on the type of addiction, but there are some common characteristics that are typically associated with addiction.

Physical signs: Physical signs of addiction can include changes in weight or appetite, changes in sleep patterns, poor hygiene, and an increase in physical illnesses or injuries. Additionally, there may be physical signs of substance use, such as bloodshot eyes, slurred speech, and track marks on the skin.

Behavioral signs: Behavioral signs of addiction can include changes in work or school performance, financial problems, legal problems, and problems with relationships. Additionally, there may be changes in patterns of substance use or engagement in addictive behaviors, such as using more of a substance or engaging in a behavior more frequently.

Emotional signs: Emotional signs of addiction can include mood swings, irritability, depression, and anxiety. Individuals with addiction may also have a lack of interest in hobbies or activities that they used to enjoy, and may become isolated from friends and family.

Cognitive signs: Cognitive signs of addiction can include changes in memory, difficulty concentrating, and problems with decision-making and impulse control.

Tolerance and withdrawal: Tolerance and withdrawal are also common symptoms of addiction. Tolerance refers to the need for more of a substance or behavior to achieve the same effects. Withdrawal refers to the physical and psychological symptoms that occur when an individual stops using a substance or engaging in a behavior.

It's important to note that not all individuals with addiction will experience all of these signs and symptoms, and that the severity and duration of these signs and symptoms can vary widely. Additionally, addiction can be a chronic disorder that can manifest differently in different individuals, and that it is important to seek professional help to diagnose and treat addiction.

Diagnosis and Assessment Tools

The diagnosis of addiction involves a comprehensive assessment that includes a medical and psychological evaluation, as well as a review of the individual's medical and family history.

Medical and Psychological Evaluation: A medical and psychological evaluation typically includes a physical examination, laboratory tests, and an interview with a healthcare professional. The healthcare professional will ask about the individual's substance use or engagement in addictive behaviors, as well as any related physical or mental health problems. They will also ask about the individual's family history of addiction and any previous treatment for addiction.

Self-report questionnaires: Self-report questionnaires are a commonly used assessment tool for addiction. These questionnaires typically ask about the individual's substance use or engagement in addictive behaviors, as well as any related physical or mental health problems. Some examples of commonly used self-report questionnaires include the CAGE questionnaire, the Alcohol Use Disorder Identification Test (AUDIT), and the Drug Abuse Screening Test (DAST).

Behavioral observation: Behavioral observation can also be used to assess addiction. This can include observing an individual's behavior in different settings, such as at work or at home, and noting any signs of substance use or engagement in addictive behaviors.

Addiction Severity Index (ASI): The Addiction Severity Index (ASI) is a widely used assessment tool that helps to identify the severity of addiction, as well as any related problems in the areas of medical, employment, legal, family/social, and psychiatric.

Interview-Based Assessment: Interview-based assessment such as the Diagnostic Interview Schedule for DSM-5 (DIS-5) or the Structured Clinical Interview for DSM-5 (SCID-5) is also used as a diagnostic tool for addiction. These assessments are conducted by trained mental health professionals, and include questions about the individual's substance use or engagement in addictive behaviors, as well as any related physical or mental health problems.

It's important to note that the diagnosis of addiction is a complex process that involves multiple steps and the use of various assessment tools. Additionally, the diagnosis of addiction should be made by a qualified healthcare professional, such as a physician, psychiatrist, or psychologist.

Differentiating Addiction from other Mental Health Conditions

Differentiating addiction from other mental health conditions can be challenging, as addiction often co-occurs with other mental health conditions and the symptoms can overlap. However, there are some key differences that can help to differentiate addiction from other mental health conditions.

Compulsion: Addiction is characterized by a compulsive engagement in a substance or behavior despite negative consequences, while other mental health conditions such as anxiety or depression are not characterized by a compulsive behavior.

Tolerance and withdrawal: Addiction is characterized by tolerance and withdrawal, which are not typically present in other mental health conditions. Tolerance refers to the need for more of a substance or behavior to achieve the same effects, and withdrawal refers to the physical and psychological symptoms that occur when an individual stops using a substance or engaging in a behavior.

Impact on daily life: Addiction can have a significant impact on an individual's daily life, including problems with work or school, finances, and relationships, while other mental health conditions such as anxiety or depression may not have such a profound impact on daily life.

Treatment: Addiction is typically treated with a combination of medications, behavioral therapies, and support groups, while other mental health conditions are treated with a combination of medications and psychotherapy.

Medical and Psychological Evaluation: A medical and psychological evaluation can help to identify the specific symptoms and characteristics of addiction, as well as any co-occurring mental health conditions.

It's important to note that addiction is a complex disorder that can manifest differently in different individuals, and that the diagnosis of addiction should be made by a qualified healthcare professional, such as a physician, psychiatrist, or psychologist. Additionally, it's important to note that co-occurring addiction and mental health disorders are common and should be treated together for a better outcome.

Treatment Options for Addiction

Medications

There are several medications that can be used to treat addiction, which can be broadly categorized into three main groups:

Medications for detoxification: These medications are used to help individuals safely and comfortably withdraw from a substance. Examples include methadone for opioid addiction, buprenorphine for opioid addiction, and naltrexone for opioid and alcohol addiction.

Medications for maintenance therapy: These medications are used to help individuals maintain abstinence from a substance, by reducing cravings and decreasing the risk of relapse. Examples include methadone and buprenorphine for opioid addiction, and naltrexone for opioid and alcohol addiction.

Medications for specific substance use disorder: Some medications are specific to treat a certain type of substance use disorder, such as varenicline for smoking cessation and acamprosate and disulfiram for alcohol addiction.

It's important to note that medication should be combined with behavioral therapy, counseling and other forms of support to achieve the best outcome. Additionally, the choice of medication will depend on the substance being used and the individual's specific needs and circumstances. The treatment should be tailored to the specific needs of the patient and monitored closely by a healthcare professional to ensure safety and effectiveness.

Behavioral Therapies

There are several behavioral therapies that can be used to treat addiction, which can be broadly categorized into three main groups:

Cognitive-behavioral therapy (CBT): This therapy aims to help individuals understand the thoughts and feelings that contribute to their addiction and to develop new coping skills to deal with these thoughts and feelings. CBT can be done individually or in a group setting.

Contingency management: This therapy uses a rewards-based system to reinforce positive behavior and discourage substance use. For example, an individual may earn vouchers or prizes for remaining abstinent from a substance, which can be exchanged for tangible goods or services.

Motivational interviewing (MI): This therapy aims to help individuals overcome ambivalence about change and to increase their motivation to change their substance use behavior. MI is a client-centered, directive method for enhancing intrinsic motivation to change by exploring and resolving ambivalence.

Family therapies: Family therapies aim to involve family members in the treatment process and to address any issues that may be contributing to the individual's addiction. Family therapy can be helpful to improve communication, problem-solving skills and emotional support.

Group therapies: Group therapies provide a supportive environment where

41

individuals can share their experiences, learn from others, and receive feedback and support. Group therapies can be helpful to increase social support, build self-esteem and reduce feelings of isolation.

It's important to note that Behavioral therapies should be individualized and tailored to the specific needs of the patient, also that treatment should be delivered by trained and qualified professionals and combined with other forms of support such as medication, counseling and self-help groups for the best outcome.

Support Groups and Self-Help

There are several support groups and self-help groups that can be used to treat addiction. These include:

12-step programs: The most well-known and widely used support groups for addiction treatment are 12-step programs, such as Alcoholics Anonymous (AA) and Narcotics Anonymous (NA). These programs are based on the idea of mutual support and include a set of principles and practices for recovery. They are designed to provide a supportive community of individuals who are also in recovery and offer a structured approach to recovery that includes regular meetings, sponsorship and working through the 12 steps.

SMART Recovery: This self-help program is based on cognitive-behavioral therapy and rational emotive behavior therapy and focuses on empowering individuals to take control of their own recovery.

Secular Organizations for Sobriety (SOS): This self-help program focuses on empowering individuals to take control of their own recovery and does not include any spiritual or religious components.

Women for Sobriety (WFS): This self-help program specifically for women who are recovering from addiction and focuses on addressing the unique challenges that women may face in recovery.

LifeRing Secular Recovery: This self-help program focuses on empowering individuals to take control of their own recovery and does not include any spiritual or religious components.

It's important to note that support groups and self-help groups can provide a valuable source of support and encouragement for individuals in recovery, but they should not be used as a sole treatment for addiction. They should be used in conjunction with other forms of treatment such as medication and behavioral therapies, and be facilitated by trained professionals. They can also serve as a supplement to the treatment, providing a network of peers in recovery, a sense of community, and a place to share experiences and receive emotional support.

Complementary and Alternative Therapies

There are several complementary and alternative therapies that can be used to treat addiction:

Mind-body therapies: These therapies aim to address the connection between the mind and the body, and can include practices such as yoga, meditation, and mindfulness. These therapies can be helpful to reduce stress and anxiety, improve emotional well-being, and promote relaxation.

Herbal and dietary supplements: Some herbal and dietary supplements may be used to help individuals manage the symptoms of addiction and withdrawal. For example, omega-3 fatty acids may be used to help reduce inflammation in the brain, and N-acetylcysteine (NAC) may be used to help reduce cravings.

Acupuncture: Acupuncture is a traditional Chinese medicine that involves the insertion of thin needles into specific points on the body. It can be helpful to reduce cravings, manage withdrawal symptoms and improve overall well-being.

Art and Music therapies: These therapies use creative and expressive techniques such as painting, drawing, dancing or music to explore and express emotions and feelings, and can be helpful to reduce stress, anxiety, and depression.

It's important to note that complementary and alternative therapies should be used in conjunction with other forms of treatment such as medication and behavioral therapies, and be facilitated by trained professionals. Also, it's important to be aware that some complementary and alternative therapies may have potential risks and side effects, and it's important to consult with a healthcare professional before starting any new therapy.

Managing Addiction in Daily Life

Coping Strategies for Cravings and Triggers

Cravings and triggers are common challenges for individuals in recovery from addiction. Coping strategies can help individuals manage cravings and triggers, and prevent relapse. Some strategies include:

Identifying triggers: One of the most effective coping strategies is to identify the triggers that lead to cravings. Triggers can be external, such as people, places or things, or internal, such as emotions or thoughts. Once triggers are identified, individuals can develop a plan to avoid or manage them.

Distraction: Engaging in activities that divert attention away from cravings can be helpful. Examples include exercise, reading, listening to music, or doing a puzzle.

Mindfulness: Mindfulness practices such as meditation or yoga can help individuals to focus on the present moment and to be aware of cravings and triggers without acting on them.

Relaxation techniques: Relaxation techniques such as deep breathing, progressive muscle relaxation, or visualization can help individuals to reduce stress and tension and to manage cravings and triggers.

Support: Having a support system in place can be beneficial in managing cravings and triggers. Support can come from friends, family, or support groups such as Alcoholics Anonymous or Narcotics Anonymous.

Self-Care: Self-care activities such as eating well, getting enough sleep, and regular exercise can help to improve overall well-being and reduce cravings and triggers.

Professional Help: Counseling or therapy can be useful to explore underlying issues that may be contributing to cravings and triggers and help to develop coping strategies.

It's important to note that coping strategies for cravings and triggers will vary from person to person, and what works for one person may not work for another. It's important for individuals in recovery to experiment with different strategies and find what works best for them. Additionally, it's also important to remember that cravings and triggers can be a normal part of the recovery process, and not to get discouraged if they occur.

Relapse Prevention

Relapse prevention is an important aspect of addiction treatment, as relapse is a common occurrence in the recovery process. Relapse prevention involves identifying and managing the risk factors that can lead to relapse, and developing a plan to prevent it. Some strategies for relapse prevention include:

Identifying high-risk situations: Identifying situations that may lead to a relapse, such as being around people who use drugs or alcohol, can help individuals to develop a plan to avoid or manage them.

Developing coping strategies: Developing coping strategies to manage cravings and triggers, such as the ones mentioned above, can help individuals to prevent relapse.

Continuing treatment: Continuing with treatment, such as therapy or medication, and attending support groups can help to prevent relapse.

Building a support network: Building a support network of friends, family, and healthcare professionals can provide a safety net and help to prevent relapse.

Staying active: Staying active in activities that promote well-being, such as exercise, hobbies, or volunteering can help to prevent relapse.

Staying mindful: Staying mindful of the warning signs of relapse, such as changes in mood or behavior, and being aware of one's own thoughts and feelings can help to prevent relapse.

Reviewing the relapse: If a relapse occurs, it's important to review the reasons and triggers that led to it, and to develop a plan to prevent it from happening again.

It's important to note that relapse prevention is a continuous process and should be considered as a part of lifelong recovery. It's also important to remember that relapse is a normal part of the recovery process, and not to get discouraged if it occurs. With the right support and strategies, individuals can prevent relapse and maintain a long-term recovery.

Building a Support System

Building a support system is an important aspect of addiction recovery, as it can provide emotional, practical and social support. Support systems can help individuals to cope with the challenges of recovery, prevent relapse and promote well-being. Some strategies for building a support system include:

Identifying supportive people: Identifying people who are supportive, understanding and non-judgmental, such as friends, family, or support groups, can help to build a support system.

Joining support groups: Joining support groups, such as 12-step programs, can provide a sense of community, and a place to share experiences, and receive emotional and practical support.

Building a relationship with a therapist or counselor: Building a relationship with a therapist or counselor can provide emotional support and help to address underlying issues that may be contributing to addiction.

Building a relationship with a physician or other healthcare professional: Building a relationship with a physician or other healthcare professional can provide medical and practical support, and help to manage withdrawal symptoms and side effects of medication.

Creating a crisis plan: Creating a crisis plan can help to prepare for high-risk situations, and provide a sense of security and control.

Self-help: Self-help resources such as books, websites, and apps can provide additional support and education.

Building a daily routine: Building a daily routine can provide structure and help to promote well-being.

It's important to note that building a support system takes time and effort, and that it's important to be patient and persistent. Also, it's important to remember that support systems can change and evolve over time, and that it's important to be open to new opportunities for support. Additionally, It's important for individuals in recovery to involve their support system in the recovery process, and to communicate their needs and expectations.

Key Takeaways

Maintaining Healthy Habits and Self-Care

Maintaining healthy habits and self-care is an important aspect of addiction recovery, as it can help to promote well-being, prevent relapse and support long-term recovery. Some strategies for maintaining healthy habits and self-care include:

Eating a healthy diet: Eating a healthy diet can help to improve overall well-being, reduce cravings and triggers, and promote a healthy weight.

Getting enough sleep: Getting enough sleep can help to reduce stress, improve mood and promote overall well-being.

Regular exercise: Regular exercise can help to reduce stress, improve mood, and promote overall well-being.

Managing stress: Managing stress through techniques such as meditation, yoga or deep breathing can help to reduce cravings and triggers, and promote overall well-being.

Practicing mindfulness: Practicing mindfulness can help to reduce stress, improve mood, and promote overall well-being.

Building a daily routine: Building a daily routine can provide structure and help to promote well-being.

Seeking help when needed: Seeking professional help when needed, such as counseling or therapy, can help to address underlying issues that may be contributing to addiction and promote overall well-being.

Avoiding risky situations: Avoiding risky situations, such as being around people who use drugs or alcohol, can help to prevent relapse and promote overall well-being.

It's important to note that maintaining healthy habits and self-care takes time and effort, and that it's important to be patient and persistent. Also, it's important to remember that what works for one person may not work for another, and that it's important to experiment with different strategies and find what works best for the individual. Additionally, it's important for individuals in recovery to involve their support system in the recovery process,

and to communicate their needs and
expectations. 64

Importance of Seeking Professional Help

Seeking professional help is an important aspect of addiction recovery, as it can provide specialized treatment and support. Professional help can include a variety of healthcare professionals such as:

Addiction specialists: Addiction specialists are healthcare professionals who are trained to provide specialized treatment for addiction. They can provide assessment, diagnosis, and treatment planning, as well as medication management, therapy, and counseling.

Psychologists and Psychiatrists: These healthcare professionals are trained to provide therapy and counseling for addiction. They can help individuals to address underlying emotional and mental health issues that may be contributing to addiction.

Medical doctors: Medical doctors can provide medical assessment, management of withdrawal symptoms and side effects of medication, and monitor overall health.

Social workers: Social workers can provide support and resources for individuals and families affected by addiction. They can help with issues such as housing, employment, and child care.

Support groups: Support groups such as 12-step programs and self-help groups can provide a sense of community, and a place to share experiences, and receive emotional and practical support.

Seeking professional help can provide a range of benefits such as:

Accurate diagnosis and treatment planning: Professional help can provide an accurate diagnosis and treatment planning that is tailored to the individual's specific needs.

Medication management: Professionals can provide medication management to help with withdrawal symptoms and reduce the risk of relapse.

Therapy and counseling: Professional therapy and counseling can help individuals to address underlying emotional and mental health issues that may be contributing to addiction and develop coping strategies for cravings and triggers.

Support and resources: Professional help can provide support and resources for individuals and families affected by addiction.

Monitoring of overall health: Professionals can monitor overall health, including any physical and psychological side effects of addiction.

It's important to note that seeking professional help is a personal decision and that it's important to find a healthcare professional that the individual feels comfortable with. Also, it's important to remember that recovery is a continuous process and that professional help should be sought as needed throughout the recovery journey.

The Stigma Around Addiction

Addiction is often stigmatized in society, which can make it difficult for individuals with addiction to seek help and recover. Stigma refers to negative attitudes, beliefs, and behaviors directed towards individuals with addiction and their families. Some of the ways that addiction is stigmatized include:

Negative stereotypes: Addiction is often associated with negative stereotypes such as laziness, weakness, and moral failing. These stereotypes can lead to discrimination and prejudice towards individuals with addiction.

Lack of understanding: Addiction is often misunderstood and seen as a choice rather than a chronic illness. This lack of understanding can lead to blame and shame for individuals with addiction and their families.

Limited access to treatment: Stigma can make it difficult for individuals with addiction to access appropriate treatment and support services. This can be due to a lack of funding or resources, as well as discrimination and prejudice from healthcare professionals.

Social isolation: Stigma can lead to social isolation for individuals with addiction, as they may be shunned by family and friends and may feel ashamed to reach out for help.

Limited representation in media: Addiction is often depicted in a negative light in the media and can reinforce stereotypes and lack of understanding.

Limited research and funding: Stigma can lead to limited research and funding for addiction treatment and support services, making it difficult for individuals with addiction to access appropriate care.

The impact of stigma on individuals with addiction can be significant, and can lead to decreased self-esteem, poor self-worth, and increased shame, guilt, and hopelessness. This can also lead to a reluctance to seek help, which can prolong the addiction, and make it harder for the individual to recover. It's important for society to become more informed and educated about addiction, so that the negative stereotypes and misconceptions are reduced and replaced with more accurate understanding and empathy.

Hope for Recovery

Recovering from addiction can be a challenging and difficult journey, but it is also a journey that is full of hope and the potential for a fulfilling life in sobriety. It's important to remember that addiction is a chronic illness, and that recovery is a continuous process that requires effort and commitment.

One of the most important things to remember is that recovery is possible. Many individuals have successfully overcome addiction and have gone on to lead fulfilling and meaningful lives in sobriety. There are many different treatment options available, such as medication, behavioral therapies, support groups and self-help groups, as well as complementary and alternative therapies that can be tailored to the individual's specific needs.

It's also important to build a strong support system, which can include friends, family, healthcare professionals and support groups. A strong support system can provide emotional, practical and social support, and can help individuals to cope with the challenges of recovery and prevent relapse.

Self-care and maintaining healthy habits are also important aspects of recovery. Eating a healthy diet, getting enough sleep, regular exercise, managing stress, practicing mindfulness and building a daily routine can help to improve overall well-being, reduce cravings and triggers, and prevent relapse.

It's important to remember that recovery is not a linear process and that setbacks are a normal part of the recovery process. It's important not to get discouraged and to keep working towards recovery. Seeking professional help when needed. and reviewing the reasons and triggers that led to setbacks and developing a plan to prevent them from happening again.

Resources for Further Information and Support

There are many resources available for further information and support for those suffering from addiction. Some of these include:

National helplines: There are several national helplines that provide information and support for individuals with addiction and their families, such as the Substance Abuse and Mental Health Services Administration (SAMHSA) National Helpline at 1-800-662-HELP (4357).

Support groups: Support groups such as Alcoholics Anonymous (AA) and Narcotics Anonymous (NA) provide a sense of community and a place to share experiences, and receive emotional and practical support.

Professional organizations: Professional organizations such as the American Society of Addiction Medicine (ASAM) and the American Association for the Treatment of Opioid Dependence (AATOD) provide information and resources for healthcare professionals and individuals with addiction.

Online resources: There are many online resources that provide information and support for individuals with addiction, such as the Addiction Resource, the National Institute on Drug Abuse (NIDA) and the Substance Abuse and Mental Health Services Administration (SAMHSA)

Local resources: Local resources such as treatment centers, counseling centers, and mental health clinics provide specialized treatment and support services for individuals with addiction.

Government resources: Government resources such as the Department of Health and Human Services (HHS) and the Center for Substance Abuse Treatment (CSAT) provide information and resources for individuals with addiction.

It's important to note that it's important to find a resource that the individual feels comfortable with and that provides the right kind of support that the individual needs. It's also important to keep in mind that different resources may work better for different individuals, so it's important to explore different options and find what works best.

About the Author

Antonio is a father of two children who he loves dearly. He has been working in the field of education for almost twenty-five years, primarily with students ages K-21. He believes that basic education around addiction is key to alleviating much of the suffering caused by the disease. The simple act of knowing what to do or who to turn to for help, could make all of the difference for those who are suffering. It is his hope that one day, every hospital and school will hand out this handbook to every patient or student, just so they have the basics to understand the disease and end the stigma around addiction. Education is truly the most powerful tool we have to transform the future.

Disclaimer

Please note that the advice provided is intended for informational purposes only and should not be taken as legal or professional advice. It is important to always seek the guidance of a qualified professional when making decisions that may have legal consequences. Additionally, it is important to use your own judgment and intuition when making any decisions, as ultimately you are responsible for the outcome. Please consult with a qualified professional before making any decisions that may have legal or other significant consequences. This disclaimer is not intended to limit or exclude any liability that may not be excluded or limited by law.

This handbook was a collaboration between the author and an open AI platform, with the sole purpose of trying to save more lives, by educating everyone who picks up this handbook on understanding and managing addiction.

First Edition: 2023
ISBN: 9798374723991

Content Feedback: Please direct all feedback to
www.handbooksforhumanity.com

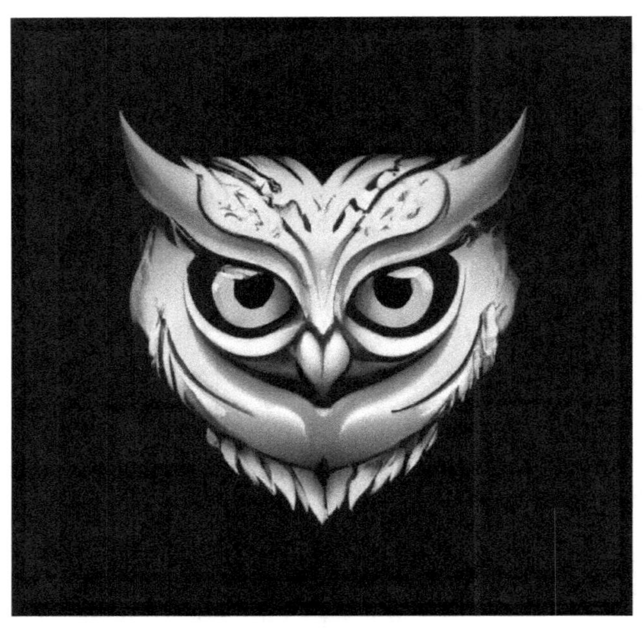

Copyright © 2023

Gufo Publishing